YOUR KNOWLEDGE HAS VALUE

AF136456

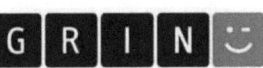

Serological Diagnostic Methods. An Overview

Isayas Asefa

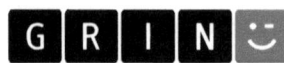

Bibliographic information published by the German National Library:

The German National Library lists this publication in the National Bibliography; detailed bibliographic data are available on the Internet at http://dnb.dnb.de.

ISBN: 9783346635907
This book is also available as an ebook.

© GRIN Publishing GmbH
Nymphenburger Straße 86
80636 München

Print and binding: Books on Demand GmbH, Norderstedt, Germany
Printed on acid-free paper from responsible sources.

The present work has been carefully prepared. Nevertheless, authors and publishers do not incur liability for the correctness of information, notes, links and advice as well as any printing errors.

GRIN web shop: https://www.grin.com/document/1192279

SOME SEROLOGICAL ANALYTIC APPROACHES AND TEST EXECUTION IN DETERMINATION OF BOVINE BRUCELLOSIS: OVERVIEW

ISAYAS ASEFA[1]

[1]School of Veterinary Medicine, DVM student, Wolaita Sodo University, P.O. Box 138, Wolaita Sodo, Ethiopia.

Inhalt

SYNOPSIS

Bovine brucellosis is an exceptionally contagious, zoonotic and financially significant bacterial disease. The point of this paper was to review accessible logical information on serological tests for the analysis of bovine brucellosis and look at their test execution in view of sensitivity (*Se*) and specificity (*Sp*) upsides of measures. The infection was portrayed by early abortion, placentitis, epididymitis, and orchitis. The clinical image of brucellosis is not pathognomonic, and the clinical history of the patient, especially the event of fetal removal, is of central symptomatic significance. Although definitive diagnosis of bovine brucellosis is finished by disconnection and distinguishing proof of the causative agents, serological tests are normally the most preferred. The host defense mechanism against Brucella can practically be partitioned into innate or nonspecific and adaptive or specific immunity. The pathogenic brucella living being has fostered a battery of instruments to sidestep or potentially regulate both innate and adaptive immune reactions in their host. Serological tests depend on the way that Brucella *abortus*, similar to other smooth Brucella, have distinctive O-polysaccharides that incite a humoral reaction with an underlying production of IgM trailed by IgG1 and IgG2/IgA. Serological techniques accessible for the analysis of bovine brucellosis incorporate the screening serological test (Milk ring test, Rose Bengal Test (RBT) and Buffered plate agglutination test (BPAT)) and corroborative serological test, which are the complement fixation test (CFT), serum agglutination test (SAT), 2-mercaptoethanol test (2ME), indirect-enzyme-linked immunosorbent assay (iELISA), and, more recently, competitive ELISA (cELISA) and *Brucella* fluorescent polarization assay (FPA). For quite a long time is no single serological test that is suitable in each and every epidemiological circumstance and 100% precise. By and large corroborative serological techniques comprise testing every serum by different tests, normally a screening trial of high responsiveness, trailed by a corroborative trial of high particularity. Therefore, the improvement of serological tests that are quick, modest, and having high awareness and explicitness for brucellosis recognition are significant issues that need further exploration.

Keywords: Bovine Brucellosis; Brucella *abortus;* diagnosis; sensitivity; specificity; serological tests, test execution.

1.   INTRODUCTION

Brucellosis is an exceptionally contagious, zoonotic and monetarily significant bacterial infection in animals worldwide (Schelling *et al.*, 2003). The disease is brought about by different types of the family Brucella, which are facultative, intracellular microscopic organisms fit for getting by and duplicating inside the cells of the mononuclear phagocytic framework (Jarvis *et al.*, 2002). The disease in cattle (bovine brucellosis), ordinarily brought about by Brucella *abortus* and sporadically by Brucella *melitensis* and Brucella *suis*, is portrayed by late-term fetus removal, infertility and diminished milk production because of held placenta and optional endometritis and discharge of the living beings in uterine releases and milk. In completely defenseless groups, early termination rates might fluctuate from 30-80% (Anonymous, 2007).

Disease is sent by dairy items such as milk, cheese and contact with contaminated animals and aerosols (Hatami *et al.*, 2010). Bovine disease presents an especially difficult issue in light of the huge volume of tainted milk that can be *developed* by a singular animal and as a result of the broad natural defilement that even single fetus removals or contaminated births can produce (Radostist *et al.*, 2000). Although developed nations have effectively controlled brucellosis, many emerging nations, for example, Ethiopia, have not had the option to respond satisfactorily, and the infection continues to be a significant public and animal medical issue. Control and annihilation of brucellosis is only in light of the serological testing of animals and the resulting winnowing of those that are seropositive for antibodies to Brucella species (OIE, 2009a).

The disease presents an extraordinary assortment of clinical indications (not pathognomonic), making it hard to analyze clinically. This shortfall of explicit indications additionally makes it difficult to separate brucellosis from a few febrile conditions that regularly occur in similar regions. Thus, the conclusion should be affirmed directly by the disengagement of Brucella, generally from blood culture, or serologically by the location of the resistance reaction against its antigens (Orduna *et al.*, 2000). Isolation and ID of causative bacterium is the best quality level for finding brucellosis; however, it requires a high security lab, profoundly talented staff, and a drawn-out pivot time for results, and it is viewed as a perilous strategy (Nielsen, 2002). In this manner, analyses are essentially founded on the identification of antibodies in serum by serological tests such as the Rapid Plate Agglutination Test (RPAT), Rose Bengal Test (RBT), Standard Agglutination Test (SAT), 2-Mercapto Ethanol Test (2ME) and Complement Fixation Test (CFT) (McGiven et al., 2003). They are moderately simple to perform and provide a pragmatic benefit in distinguishing the predominance of Brucella disease (Abubakar et al., 2011).

Body liquids, for example, serum, uterine release, vaginal bodily fluid and milk or semen plasma from associated cattle, might contain various amounts of antibodies of the IgM, IgG1, IgG2 and IgA types coordinated against Brucella (OIE, 2000). Antibodies as a rule show up in the blood toward the end of the principal seven-day stretch of the disease, IgM showing up first followed by IgG (Lucero et al., 2003). Accordingly, serological techniques are prescribed to obtain quick roundabout confirmation of the conclusion. Each test has its own inconveniences, and the presence of antibodies does not generally allude to the presence of a functioning brucellosis contamination (Clavijo et al., 2003).

Several serological methods are currently available; these tests can be classified as screening tests (e.g., buffered antigen plate agglutination (BPAT), Rose Bengal plate test (RBPT), monitoring or epidemiological surveillance tests (e.g., milk ring test), and complementary or confirmatory tests (e.g., 2-mercapto-ethanol, complement fixation, ELISAs, and fluorescence polarization assay). Selection of a given test should take into account the species affected as well as local regulations (Poester et al., 2010). Hence, the targets of this survey paper are as follows:

➢ To survey serological analytic tests accessible for the diagnosis of Brucella diseases in bovine and

➢ To look at test execution of the accessible serological analytic tests in view of the sensitivity and specificity values.

2. HOST IMMUNE RESPONSES IN BRUCELLA INFECTION

Practically, the host insusceptible reaction is isolated into inborn or *nonspecific* and adaptive `or specific immunity (Parkin and C-ohen, 2001). Disease with Brucella ordinarily brings about the acceptance of both humoral and cell-intervened insusceptible reactions; however, the size and span of these reactions is impacted by different elements, including the destructiveness of the contaminating strain, the size of the tainting inoculum, pregnancy, and the sexual and immune status of the host (skendros, 2013).

The procedure of Brucella *abortus* is to avoid the inborn safe framework and continue in the host to the point of being communicated. The bacterium contains a strange lipid A comprising the LPS atom, which is significant for avoiding the host immune framework during the beginning phases of disease (Parent *et al.*, 2007). The variation to live inside macrophages is overseen by its capacity to obstruct receptors for natural resistance, repress phagolysosome combination, hinder apoptosis, and downregulate antigen show, which aggregately prompts their break from effector immune reactions (Martirosyan and Gorvel, 2013).

2.1. Innate Immunity

Natural immunity is a fast, nonspecific, and nonmemory safe reaction against attacking Brucella microbes. It comprises actual boundaries at the outer layer of the body, humoral parts *such as complement* proteins, and cell parts that incorporate macrophages, dendritic cells, granulocytes (basophils, eosinophils, and neutrophils) and normal executioner cells (Dranoff, 2004).

2.1.1. Physical boundaries

The body's actual boundaries give the primary degree of security and incorporate the skin and furthermore the body's 'self-cleaning' cycles, such as sniffling or hacking. Nonetheless, actual hindrances cannot be totally compelling, and some of the time, microbes might defeat them. Thus, animals have an insusceptible framework including an organization of cells and atoms that can battle contamination (Tigard, 2013).

2.1.2. Humoral parts

Complement is a foundational plasma protein with an assortment of capacities that incorporate opsonization by restriction to antibodies or bacterial surfaces or direct killing of Brucella microbes by the arrangement of a film assault complex, causing bacterial lysis (Tigard, 2012).

2.1.3. Cellular parts

Macrophages and dendritic cells are the main cells that respond to attacking organisms and are responsible for acceptance of the Adaptive immune reaction by the introduction of antigen epitopes to T partner (Th) cells. Microorganism acknowledgment is accomplished by design acknowledgment receptors (PRRs) communicated by the antigen introducing cells that perceive pathogen-associated atomic examples (PAMPs) of the attacking organisms (Pasquevich *et al.*, 2010). Bovine normal executioner cells might act straightforwardly through the discharge of IFNc, which is a cytokine that animates the bactericidal movement of macrophages (Oliveira *et al.*, 2002). Neutrophils experience and kill microorganisms intracellularly upon phagocytosis, when their antimicrobial granules meld with the phagosome. Moreover, they discharge lytic proteins and responsive oxygen species (ROS) that annihilate microbes (Nauseef, 2007).

2.2. Adaptive Immunity

The second blockade in the host arm is adaptive resistance, which is also called an antigen-explicit insusceptible reaction or explicit immunity. It comprises T lymphocytes, which are liable for cytokine *production* and cytotoxicity, known as cell-mediated immunity (CMI), and B lymphocytes, which are liable for counteracting agent *production,* known as humoral invulnerability or neutralizer intervened immunity (AMI) (Parkin and Cohen, 2001).

2.2.1. Antibody-induced resistance (AMI)

The B lymphocytes oversee the humoral arm of *Adaptive* resistance, portrayed by *production* of antigen-explicit antibodies. Notwithstanding their killing impact, antibodies go about as opsonins that work with the phagocytosis of microorganisms by antigen-introducing cells, enact complement and advance counteracting agents subordinate cell-intervened cytotoxicity (ADCC) by macrophages, neutrophils and regular executioner cells (Baldwin and Goenka, 2006). The presence of hostile to Brucella antibodies suggests openness to Brucella spp.; however, it does not demonstrate which Brucella species incited the production of those antibodies. Tainted animals may not dependably produce all counteracting agent isotypes in perceptible amounts; consequently, the results from a few serological tests ought to be utilized as a hypothetical proof of disease (FAO, 2005).

The neutralizer reaction to Brucella *abortus* in dairy cattle comprises the early *production* of IgM, and it very quickly advances to the development of IgG2 and later delivers limited quantities of IgG1 and IgA (Goenka *et al.*, 2012). Thus, the presence of IgM demonstrates an early immune reaction (intense disease) against brucellosis, and IgG correspondingly shows persistent contamination or backslides. It is notable that enemies of Brucella antibodies can possibly cross-respond with antibodies raised against heterologous Brucella strains or against a few intestinal microorganisms. This cross-reactivity hampered the understanding of large numbers of serological tests utilized in the analysis of brucellosis (Young, 2005).

2.2.2. Cell-mediated immunity (CMI)

Bunch differentiation (CD4) and group differentiation (CD8) T cells have been shown to play a role in adaptive resistant reactions to Brucella (Carvalho *et al.*, 2010). T helper cells are CD4+ cells and incorporate T aide type 1 (Th1) and T aide type 2 (Th2) that act essentially as partner cells for cell-mediated inflammatory responses, for example, deferred extreme hypersensitivity and macrophage initiation, and stimulate counteracting agent production, especially IgE, IgG1, and IgA. Cytotoxic lymphocytes (CTLs) kill target cells basically through two significant pathways: First, the Fas ligand on CTLs interacts with its Fas receptor on track cells and then enacts a self-destruction pathway in the target cells; and second, the CTLs exocytose granules containing perforin and granzymes that structure pores in target cell film and possibly cause cell death (Janeway at el, 2001).

3. SEROLOGICAL DIAGNOSTIC TESTS IN BOVINE BRUCELLOSIS

Serological tests have a long history and have been utilized effectively for the diagnosis of many infectious diseases (e.g., HIV, syphilis, and viral hepatitis) (Steingart *et al.*, 2012). Serological symptomatic tests for brucellosis have been developed over a century prior; in any case, the ideal test has still not been developed. Customary serological techniques for Brucella diagnostics depend on the identification of antibodies, explicit to the surface LPS (He, 2012)

Serological tests are critical for laboratorial finding of brucellosis since a large portion of control and annihilation projects of brucellosis rely upon these techniques. Inactivated entire microorganisms or cleaned divisions (for example, lipopolysaccharide or film proteins) are utilized as antigens for distinguishing antibodies produced by the host during

9

contamination. Antibodies against smooth Brucella species (for example, B. *abortus,* B. *melitensis,* and B. *suis*) cross-respond with antigen arrangements from B. *abortus,* although antibodies against unpleasant Brucella species (for example, B. *ovis* and B. *canis)* cross-respond with antigen arrangements from B. *ovis* (Nielsen, 2002).

Serological tests are conservative and dependable instruments of finding as there is a decent relationship between disconnection of Brucella and positive tests performed with sera and milk. When tests for identifying Brucella antibodies in milk and serum are considered, the key strategies for distinguishing tainted groups and for diagnosing brucellosis in individual animals are serological tests, which are mostly utilized for finding brucellosis (Noriello, 2004).

The decision of the serological symptomatic technique relies upon the general epidemiological circumstances in the district and the goals of the review: approval of the conclusion, screening (observing), cross-sectional investigations or affirmation of the SARS brucellosis status of the locale (Godfroid *et al.,* 2010). Test result translation ought to consistently consider the accompanying components: percentage of positive test results, disease pervasiveness and frequency; presence of clinical signs (fetus removal); inoculation system; realized danger factors; status of the group, the region, and the country (European Commission, 2009). The awareness and explicitness of serological tests have been viewed as affected by the outside climate, for example, the temperature conditions under which the test is played out, the infection endemic status, animal immunization and the presence of cross-responding antibodies from other Gram-negative microscopic organisms that share comparable epitopes with Brucella species. Although a few serological tests have been utilized for the research center testing of brucellosis, no single test is helpful in all epidemiological examinations because of issues of responsiveness and particularity (Matope *et al.,* 2011). There are a few serological methods that can be utilized relying upon the antibodies being contemplated (Ryan and Ray, 2004). They can be extensively partitioned into two gatherings: screening tests and corroborative tests (FAO, 2003). Among them, ELISA is the most touchy and explicit of the Brucella serologic routine tests and is valuable to screen antibodies in patients going

10

through treatment, isotype deciding and period of infection, and it very well might be positive when different tests are negative (Esmaeilzadeh, 2004).

3.1. Screening Serological Tests

Screening tests are quick and reasonable techniques with high aversion to guarantee that contaminated animals are not missed. It is recommended that all animals in a tainted crowd, including those that test negative during screening, be progressively assessed utilizing corroborative tests (Adone and Pasquali, 2013). There are many screening tests that are utilized to analyze brucellosis in bovines. A few screening tests utilized in the field facilities or in provincial labs are the Rose Bengal test, Buffered Plate Agglutination Test (BPAT), and Milk Ring test (MRT). The Rose Bengal Plate Test (RBPT) is the most widely recognized serological test for the discovery of Brucella agglutinins. The Rose Bengal Plate Test (RBPT) has an extremely high aversion to guarantee that contaminated animals are not missed. The milk ring test is likewise a magnificent evaluating test for dairy cows (FAO, 2003).

3.1.1. Rose-Bengal plate test (RBT)

The Rose-Bengal Test (RBT) is the most conservative and most broadly utilized research center test in the determination of bovine brucellosis; however, the understanding of the outcome is generally abstract (Konstantinidis 2007). It is a quick, slide-type agglutination measure performed with a stained B. *abortus* suspension at pH 3.6-3.7 and plain serum. However, the low pH (3.6) of the antigen improves the explicitness of the test and temperature of the antigen, and the encompassing temperature at which the response occurs may impact the responsiveness and particularity of the test (AUSVETPLAN, 2005). The awareness is exceptionally high (>99%), yet the explicitness is disappointingly as low as 68.8% (Barrsol et al., 2002). Be that as it may, this is of worth as a screening test in high danger rustic regions where it is preposterous all of the time to play out the cylinder agglutination titration test (Mantur et al., 2006).

11

Its effortlessness made it an optimal evaluating test for small labs with restricted assets. The rule of the test is that the sera gathered from animals that were removed at -20°C were removed from the cooler and left at room temperature for no less than 30 minutes before the test was performed. For this test, 30 mL of plain serum was administered on a white reflexive clay tile and blended with an equivalent volume of RBT antigen (recently equilibrated at room temperature and shaken to resuspend any bacterial dregs) utilizing a toothpick. The tile is then shaken at room temperature for 4 minutes (rather than the 8 minutes suggested for human brucellosis), and any apparent agglutination as well as the presence of an ordinary edge is taken as a positive outcome (Araj, 1999).

The Rose Bengal plate test (RBPT) is the most generally involved evaluating test for brucellosis in the two people and animals for its simple application and obvious effortlessness of perusing. Nevertheless, translations of the RBPT results can be impacted by private experience (Cho *et al.*, 2010). The downsides of RBT include low awareness, especially in ongoing cases, generally low particularity in endemic regions and prozones, making firmly certain sera seem negative in RBT (Diaz, 2011).

In cows, in regions where there is almost no disease and especially where there has been many strain 19 immunization, the RBPT-positive sera must be exposed to corroborative tests. In vigorously tainted crowds, it might be conservative to eliminate all animals positive to this test, since numerous such animals, albeit negative to corroborative tests, might be in the beginning phases of contamination and liable to become risky in spreading brucellosis later (Brinley *et al.*, 1996). Negative bogus responses happen in the RBT; nonetheless, these tests are considered reasonable evaluating tests for brucellosis, trailed by corroborative testing. The immune response coming about because of Brucella *abortus* s19 inoculation will respond in these tests (OIE, 2008).

3.1.2. Milk ring test (MRT)

The milk ring test (MRT) is a basic and compelling serological technique; however, it must be utilized with cow's milk. A drop of hematoxylin-stained antigen is blended with a small volume of milk in a glass or plastic cylinder. Assuming explicit immunizer is available in the milk, it will tie to the antigen and ascend with the cream to shape a blue ring at the highest point of the segment of milk. On the off chance that no neutralizer is available, the fat layer will stay a buff tone (the cream stays boring), and the purple antigen will be disseminated all through the milk. This test might be applied to individual animals or to pooled milk tests utilizing a larger volume of milk compared with the pool size. The test is sensibly delicate; however, it may neglect to identify a few tainted animals inside a large crowd. Nonspecific responses are normal with this test, particularly in brucellosis-free regions (Corbel *et al.*, 2006).

At present, veterinary analytic research facilities use the milk ring test for the analysis of brucellosis in bovine milk tests, which in a roundabout way distinguishes Brucella species in the host (Chimana *et al.*, 2010). The Brucella milk ring test can be utilized for screening the crowd and to show the level of disease in a group. The test can be applied to screen the dairy groups at standard stretches. Although moderately modest and simple to play out, this test does not give exact outcomes. There is a high level of bogus positive outcomes. Critically, the quantity of bogus positive outcomes corresponds to the quantity of cows emitting acidic milk because of colostrums or mastitis (OIE, 2009).

The milk ring test is inclined to bogus responses made by strange milk due to mastitis, the presence of colostrum and milk from late lactation. All things considered, despite these issues, might be utilized as an economical screening test related to different tests (Fernando *et al.*, 2010). This test is not viewed as delicate; however, this absence of responsiveness is remunerated by the way that the test can be rehashed, generally month to month, because of its exceptionally minimal expense. This test is recommended by the OIE for utilization with cow milk alone (OIE, 2009)

13

3.1.3. Buffered plate agglutination test

Buffered plate agglutination (BPA) tests are notable supported Brucella antigen tests. These tests are fast agglutination tests lasting 4 minutes and are performed on a glass plate with the assistance of an acidic-supported antigen (pH 3.65 ± 0.05). These tests have been presented in numerous nations as the standard screening test since they are extremely straightforward and thought to be more delicate than the SAT (Greiner *et al.*, 2009). In BPAT, the cells are stained with Crystal Violet and suspended in a cradle, which, when blended with a suitable volume of serum, brings about a final pH of 3.65. This PH reduces agglutination by IgM but supports agglutination by IgG1, diminishing the cross response. Counteracting agent coming about because of B. *abortus* s19 inoculation will respond in these tests. These tests are considered an appropriate evaluating test for brucellosis followed by corroborative tests such as CFT (Miguel *et al.*, 2011).

3.2. Confirmatory serological tests

The corroborative serological test is a test that gives great awareness, however, higher test particularity, subsequently removing a few bogus positive responses. All screening test results that show positive experimental outcomes should be confirmed by corroborative serological tests, as there are positive experimental outcomes for bogus. Most corroborative tests are muddled and costly to perform (Fernando *et al.*, 2010). There are numerous serological tests that can be utilized as corroborative serological tests for bovine brucellosis. Among them, the most widely recognized are the Complement Fixation Test (CFT), Enzyme Linked Immune Sorbent Assay (ELISA), Serum Agglutination Test (SAT), 2-mercaptoethanol test (2MT), Fluorescence polarization examine (FPA) and Brucellin allergic skin test (BAST). Among them, ELISA and CFT are the most ordinarily utilized corroborative serological tests (FAO, 2003).

3.2.1. Complement fixation test

The complement obsession test is a broadly involved corroborative test for brucellosis. The essential test comprises B. *abortus* antigen, typically entire cells, hatched with weakening of hotness inactivated (to obliterate native complement) serum and titrated wellspring of complement, for the most part guinea pig serum (Gupte and Kaur, 2015). It is the best quality level test for serological conclusion of brucellosis in cows (OIE, 2009). The Complement Fixation Test (CFT) permits the recognition of against Brucella antibodies that can enact complement. Cows immunoglobulins (Ig) that can enact bovine complement are IgG and IgM. The CFT test is profoundly explicit, yet it requires exceptionally prepared faculty just as reasonable research center offices. It estimates a larger number of antibodies of the IgG1 type than antibodies of the IgM type (Nielson, 2001).

The test depends on the rule that initiation of the complement framework by antigen-counteracting agent edifices within the sight of red platelets will prompt hemolysis of red platelets, which can be assessed outwardly. Complement in the test serum is heat inactivated before the expansion of the entire cell Brucella CFT antigen and hatching to permit the complement course to happen if hostile to Brucella antibodies are available supposed *complement* obsession (Au IBAR, 2013).

The Complete obsession test is generally utilized and acknowledged as a corroborative test although it is perplexing to perform, requiring great lab offices and enough prepared staff to precisely titrate and keep up with the reagents (Xavler *et al.*, 2009). The responsiveness of complement obsession ranges from 77.1 to 100 percent, and its explicitness ranges from 65 to 100 percent (Perrett *et al.*, 2010). It is exceptionally proficient and, in this manner, acknowledged around the world (Nielsen, 2002).

The Complement obsession test is actually difficult in light of the fact that countless reagents should be titrated day by day and countless controls of the relative multitude of reagents are required. It is likewise a costly test again as a result of the huge number of reagents required and on the grounds that it is work escalated. Since only the IgG1 isotype of the neutralizer fixes complement well, the test explicitness is high. Unfortunately, the test does not take into consideration segregation of B. *abortus* s19 inferred neutralizer. Different issues incorporate the subjectivity of the translation of results, periodic direct actuation of complement by serum (anticomplementary action) and the powerlessness of the test for use with hemolysed serum tests. Disregarding the inadequacies, the Complement obsession test has been and is an important resource as a corroborative test in charge/destruction projects of brucellosis (Fernando *et al.*, 2010).

3.2.2. 2-Mercaptoethanol (2ME) test

2-Mercaptoethanol (2ME) is a corroborative serological test that permits particular measurement of IgG against Brucella because of inactivation of IgM in the test. Production of IgG is normally connected with constant contamination, and along these lines, a positive outcome with this test is a solid mark of brucellosis. In any case, this test has a few downsides, including the poisonousness of mercaptoethanol, which requires a smoke hood for its control, and the chance of IgG debasement brought about by 2-mercaptoethanol, which might bring about adverse outcomes. The test gauges primarily IgG on the grounds that the di-sulphide extension of IgM is being diminished to monometric particles and, hence, incapable of agglutinating. Notwithstanding, immunoglobulin (IgG) can likewise be decreased simultaneously, giving bogus adverse outcomes. However, as a rule, a decrease in IgM builds particularity (Poester *et al.*, 2010).

The 2-mercaptoethanol (2-ME) test can be utilized to foresee the course of the disease (Aliskan, 2008). The responsiveness of the 2-mercaptoethanol test differs from 88.4 and 99.6%, and its explicitness ranges from 91.5 and 99.8% (Nielsen, 2004). The test does not dispose of vaccinal antibodies, in this way is not suggested for global exchange. 2-MET is, notwithstanding, utilized broadly for public control as well as destruction programs (Nielsen, 2002).

3.2.3. Enzyme-connected immunosorbent assay (ELISA)

The enzyme-connected immunosorbent test is a quick serological analytic test and has a high responsiveness and explicitness of approximately 80% for the finding of IgM, IgG and IgA antibodies connected with Brucella in blood (Kostoula *et al.*, 2002). It depends on the rule that, as its name recommends, it utilizes a protein framework to show the particular blend of an antigen with its neutralizer. The protein framework comprises a compound that is marked or connected to a particular counteracting agent or antigen and a substrate that is added after the antigen immune response. This substrate is followed up on (typically hydrolyzed) by the chemical joined to the antigen immunizer buildings to give a shading change. The force of the shading gives a sign of how much antigen or antibody is bound (Beker and Kedir, 2008). This test can analyze a fragmented counteracting agent, and this immune response is for the most part detectable in constant patients with brucellosis, suggesting that this test should be used for such patients (Ertek *et al.*, 2006).

The enzyme-connected immunosorbent assay (ELISA) technique represents an extraordinary chance of ID of all four immunizer classes (IgM, IgG1, IgG2 and IgA) (Crowther, 2010). Although the ELISA procedure is viewed as perhaps the most delicate serological test and is a valuable technique for checking antibodies in patients going through treatment, the absence of a standard antigen, the varieties in the nature of arrangements and the utilization of different endpoints make the translation of ELISA results *troublesome (Clavijo et al.,* 2003). There are essentially two various types of immunoenzymatic articles that are utilized for the determination of brucellosis in people and homegrown animal species: circuitous ELISA (ELISAi) and competitive ELISA (ELISAc) (DiFebo *et al.*, 2012).

The roundabout enzyme-connected immunosorbent test is an exceptionally delicate and explicit test that can be adjusted to handle countless examples in a brief time frame, and they are conservative as long as time and exertion, with awareness and explicitness running between 98 and close to 100% for both serum and milk ELISA (OIE, 2004). The backhanded ELISA (iELISA) technique depends on the particular restriction of antibodies

17

present in the test with immobilized antigen. The restricting occasion is imagined utilizing artificially or enzymatically inferred fluorescent, radiant or colorimetric response demonstrative of the presence of immunizer in the example. Numerous iELISA tests are available (Poester et al., 2010). Aberrant ELISA for the most part has extremely high responsiveness, but since they are to a great extent unfit to recognize the B. abortus S19 vaccine immune response and cross-responding neutralizer, the particularity can be marginally lower than the test explicitness in regions where immunization is not polished (Fernando et al., 2010).

The competitive enzyme-connected immunosorbent assay (cELISA) depends on the relocation of serum antibodies by a decent grouping of a mouse monoclonal neutralizer (MAb) against the normal (C/Y) epitope, which is the prevailing epitope in the O polysaccharides of both B. abortus and B. melitensis and is the most important in serological conclusion. Since cELISA does not include the utilization of an aspecific form hostile to animal species immunoglobulin, this examination can be effectively adjusted to recognize Brucella diseases in various animal species. This cELISA utilizes SLPS latently immobilized on the mass of 96-well polystyrene plates. A contest between a monoclonal immune response explicit for a typical epitope of OPS and test serum, both suitably weakened, is added. The monoclonal immunizer might be marked straightforwardly with chemical or an auxiliary enemy of mouse counteracting agent named with compound might be added (Thompson et al., 2009). It is fit for recognizing inoculated animals or animals tainted with cross-responding organic entities from normally contaminated animals, in this manner diminishing the quantity of bogus positive reactions (OIE, 2009).

3.2.4. Serum agglutination test

The serum agglutination test is a standard serological screening test utilized for the determination of brucellosis (Memish and Balkhy, 2004). It is a serological test developed by Wright, and partners remain the most famous but involved overall analytic apparatus for the finding of brucellosis since it is not difficult to perform and does not require costly supplies and preparation. SAT estimates the complete amount of agglutinating IgM and

18

IgG antibodies. This test depends on the reactivity of antibodies against the smooth lipopolysaccharide of Brucella. Abundance of antibodies bringing about a negative bogus response due to prozone impact can be overwhelmed by applying a sequential weakening of 1:2 through 1:64 of the serum tests, accordingly expanding the test particularity (Afify *et al.*, 2013)

The amount of explicit still up in the air by treatment of the serum with 0.05 M 2-mercaptoethanol (2ME) inactivates the agglutin capacity of IgM. SAT titers above 1:160 are viewed as indicative related to a viable clinical show. Notwithstanding, in areas of endemic infection, utilizing a titer of 1:320 as a cut off may make the test more explicit. The separation in the sort of counteracting agent is additionally significant, as IgG antibodies are viewed as a preferable marker of dynamic disease over IgM, and the quick fall in the degree of IgG antibodies is supposed to be prognostic of fruitful treatment along these lines. The serum agglutination test has low awareness (41%), while its explicitness was 66.7% in bovines (Akhtar *et al.*, 2010).

3.2.5. Fluorescence polarization test

The fluorescence polarization test (FPA) is a basic procedure for estimating antigen/counteracting agent cooperation and might be performed in a research facility setting or in the field. It is a homogeneous animal type-free examination in which analytes are not isolated, and it is in this way an extremely quick test for the finding of Brucella disease (Corbel and MacMillan, 2000). The FPA was first developed for testing serum. Nonetheless, the innovation has been stretched out to testing entire blood and milk tests from individual animals (Supriya *et al.*, 2010). It depends on the actual standard of the mass-subordinate difference in the particle revolution speed in a fluid medium. The more modest the atom is, the quicker it pivots, and the depolarization of a captivated light emission occurs. In FPA, the serum test is hatched with a particular Brucella antigen, formed with a fluorescent name. In the event that there are against Brucella antibodies in the serum, a large fluorescently named antigen-neutralizer complex is framed, which can without much of a stretch be recognized from the unbound antigen negative control

(McGiven *et al.*, 2003). Hence, the revolution of a fluorescent particle (fluorophore) formed to the Brucella O-chain will slow whenever limited by hostility to Brucella LPS antibodies (Montagnaro *et al.*, 2007). Assuming serum contains antibodies to antigen, there is a reduction in the pace of pivot because of an expansion in the subatomic load of the antigen neutralizer complex. It is this abatement that empowers the differentiation between negative and positive outcomes (OIE Terrestrial Manual, 2009).

The responsiveness of the fluorescence polarization test differs from 87.5 and 100 percent, and the explicitness ranges from 84 to 100 percent (Godfread *et al.*, 2010). It is extremely precise and aware: explicitness can be controlled by modifying the cutoff esteem among positive and negative responses to give an exceptionally delicate screening test just as a profoundly explicit corroborative test. Since just 2 reagents, antigen and diluent cradle, are required, the test is actually basic and moderately cheap. It requires a fluorescence polarization analyzer, of which a few are accessible at different expenses. Demonstrative packs are likewise economically accessible from a few sources. The FPA is fit for recognizing the vaccinal immune response in most immunized animals, and it can kill a few cross responses as well (Nielsen, 2002).

Because of brucellosis serology, the small subatomic weight subunit of OPS is named fluoroescein isothiocyanate and utilized as the antigen. When testing serum, blood, or milk, assuming that neutralizer to the OPS is available, the pace of pivot of the marked antigen will be diminished. The pace of decrease is relative to how much immune response is present (Montagnaro, 2008).

3.2.6. Brucellin hypersensitive skin test

The skin test is a hypersensitivity test that distinguishes the particular cell-resistant reaction induced by Brucella contamination. The infusion of brucellergene, a protein concentrate of an unpleasant strain of Brucella species, is trailed by a neighborhood incendiary reaction in a sharpened animal. This postponed type excessive touchiness response is estimated by the increment in skin thickness at the site of inoculation. Ten square centimeters of solid clean skin on the side of the neck was shaved with scissors or electric trimmers. A tuberculin needle with a 4 mm needle was utilized to infuse 100 μl of brucellin intradermally, and the response was perused three days after the infusion. Palpation of the infusion site was the essential method for assessing the response. The apparent or potentially substantial response was evaluated by estimating the breadth of the expanding. A spring meter (Aesculap) was utilized to look at the distinction in skin thickness at the infusion site with an overlay of solid skin near the site. Skin thickening of 1.5-2 mm would be considered a positive response (Saegerman *et al.*, 1999).

The brucellin skin test has an extremely high particularity, with the end goal that serologically bad unvaccinated animals that are positive reactors to the brucellin test ought to be viewed as tainted animals (Neilsen and Yu, 2010a). Therefore, this test could be utilized as a corroborative test on dairy cattle not immunized against brucellosis. Not all contaminated animals respond; subsequently, this test alone cannot be suggested as the sole symptomatic test or for the motivations behind worldwide exchange. This test is endorsed as an elective test by the OIE (2009).

3.2.7. Rivanol plate test

The test is pointed toward dispensing with a few *nonspecific* responses that depend on precipitation of high subatomic weight serum glycoprotein from serum arrangements, which for this situation is basically IgM, leaving IgG in the serum for the most part (Montasser *et al.*, 2011). Acrydine color, for example, rivanol (2-ethoxy-6,9-diaminoacridine lactate), is utilized to accomplish the precipitation interaction, after which the hasten is removed by centrifugation. The supernatant was tested using a quick plate agglutination test with undiluted serum or a cylinder test utilizing serum weakenings of 1:25, 1:50, 1:100, and 1:200. Precipitation tests are normally utilized as corroborative tests in view of their difficult conventions (Poiester *et al.*, 2010).

3.2.8. Antiglobulin or Coomb's test

The Coomb's test is the most appropriate and touchy test for affirmation of backsliding patients with determined disease (Supriya *et al.*, 2010). The Coombs test is helpful for antibody discovery, similar to the impeding of IgG in patients who are experiencing the persistent type of infection (Galinska and Zagorski, 2013). The presence of a square on an immunizer or Prozone peculiarity causes bogus negative SAT outcomes, and subsequently, the use of the Coombs test is an optimal strategy to overcome this issue. In brucellosis finding, the SAT test is the most dependable test, yet in certain patients who have clear clinical manifestations and negative SAT outcomes, it is smarter to utilize the Coombs and chemical connected immunosorbent examination (ELISA) strategies (Serra and Vinas, 2004).

3.2.9. Native hapten and poly B tests

Local hapten and poly B tests are corroborative tests that have been utilized effectively in a destruction program in mix with the RBT as a screening test (Carrasco, 1995). The conjunctival inoculation (both in youthful and grown-ups) decreases the opportunity to acquire a negative reaction in local hapten tests. An astounding quality of the spiral immunodiffusion test is that a positive outcome corresponds with Brucella shedding in tentatively contaminated cows and in normally tainted dairy cattle going through anti-infection treatment (Joint FAO/WHO Expert Committee on Brucellosis, 1986). Precipitin tests utilizing local hapten or Brucella cytosol proteins have likewise been displayed to dispense with, much of the time, FPSR responses brought about by Yersinia enterocolitica O:9 and FPSR of obscure beginning (Munoz *et al.*, 2005).

4. TEST PERFORMANCE AND COST COMPARISON OF SEROLOGICAL TESTS

The serological tests accessible in bovine brucellosis show various exhibitions under various conditions. The demonstrative presentation of an examination is shown by the indicative responsiveness and particularity, which is characterized in the OIE Terrestrial manual as follows: Diagnostic awareness is the extent of tests from known tainted reference animals that test positive in a test. Analytic explicitness is the extent of tests from known uninfected reference animals that test negative in a test (OIE, 2013).

The awareness in the singular animal might be affected by the phase of disease or immunity of the host and the blend of cases tried. Analytic explicitness might be impacted by the presence of maternal antibodies, constancy of antibodies after recuperation or inoculation relying upon reason for testing. The responsiveness can be assessed as the genuine upsides, partitioned by the number of genuine upsides and bogus negatives. A few techniques can be utilized to decide the demonstrative exhibition of an examination. Ordinarily, demonstrative responsiveness and particularity are determined by testing tests from animals with known status (Greiner and Gardner, 2000). One more technique to gauge demonstrative responsiveness and explicitness without even a trace of information about the genuine disease status requires the utilization of muddled factual ideas and equations. It depends on the utilization of two tests, where the symptomatic awareness of one test is blemished, however known, or the responsiveness and particularity of the two tests are unknown (Enoe *et al.*, 2000).

The *complement* obsession test (CFT) is analytically more explicit than the SAT and furthermore has a normalized arrangement of unitage. The demonstrative presentation qualities of some protein connected immunosorbent measures and the fluorescence polarization examination (FPA) are practically identical to or better than those of the CFT, and as they are actually less complex to perform and stronger, their utilization might be liked (Wright *et al.*, 1997). An examination with the SAT and ELISA yields higher awareness and particularity. ELISA is likewise answered to be the touchiest test for the

23

conclusion of focal sensory system brucellosis. The symptomatic awareness and particularity of the FPA for bovine brucellosis are practically indistinguishable from those of the cELISA. Among the more upto-date serologic tests, the ELISA gives off an impression of being the touchiest; nonetheless, more experience is required before it replaces the SAT as the trial of decision for brucellosis (Almunneef and Memish, 2003).

Generally, screening tests are modest, quick and profoundly touchy, yet at the same time not truly exceptionally explicit. Corroborative tests need to be both delicate and explicit. Obviously, no single test is skilled to distinguish all sure instances of Brucella tainted animals because of variety in responsiveness and particularity of serological tests (*Salama et al.*, 2011).

Responsiveness and explicitness ranges for the normally utilized serological tests are organized beneath. These are values obtained from a few sources in the writing (Nielsen, 2002). The Performance Index gives a general gauge of the exactness of the test by adding the responsiveness and particularity esteems. In Table 2, the Min and Max esteems address the most minimal and most elevated files.

Table 1: Sensitivity, specificity and performance index of the normally involved serological tests for bovine brucellosis.

Serological Test	% Sensitivity	% Specificity	Performance Index (Min - Max)
SAT	29.1 – 100	99.2 – 100	128.3 - 200
RBT	21.0 - 98.3	68.8 – 100	89.8 - 198.3
BPAT	75.4 - 99.9	90.6 – 100	166.0 - 199.9
RIV	50.5 – 100	21.9 – 100	72.4 - 200
2ME	56.2 – 100	99.8 – 100	156.0 - 200

CFT	23.0 - 97.0	30.6 – 100	53.6 - 197.0
iELISA	92.0 – 100	90.6 – 100	182.6 - 199.8
cELISA	97.5 – 100	99.7 - 99.8	197.3 - 199.8
FPA	99.0 - 99.3	96.9 – 100	195.9 - 199.3

Source: (Nielsen, 2002), Based on a meta-examination of sensitivity (Se) and specificity (Sp) values from a few sources distributed in peer surveyed diaries, particularly diaries of animal and veterinary science.

5. ENDS AND RECOMMENDATIONS

The utilization and comprehension of various serological tests for the determination of bovine brucellosis under various conditions is important because of the confounded idea of the disease and its inborn and obtained resistance reaction. The Rose Bengal (RB) test and the Complement obsession (CF) test are the most generally involved tests for the serological determination of bovine brucellosis. There is no single serological test that is suitable in all epidemiological circumstances; all have limits, particularly with regard to screening individual animals. Despite these limits, serologic symptomatic tests are exceptionally helpful in diagnosing bovine brucellosis in dairy cattle. In all cases, a blood test ought to be gathered from the patient, and research facility testing ought to be mentioned, as the unequivocal determination of brucellosis is inconceivable without lab affirmation.

For the reasons for this audit:

> The serological techniques portrayed address normalized and approved strategies with appropriate execution attributes to be assigned as either recommended or

elective tests for global exchange. This does not block the utilization of adjusted or comparative test strategies or the utilization of various organic reagents.

➢ Doubtlessly the answer for the issues with precise serological analysis of bovine brucellosis will include a few tests for various elements of the host insusceptible reaction.

6. REFERENCES

Abubakar M., Mansoor M., and Arshed M.J. (2011): Bovine Brucellosis. Old and new concepts with Pakistan perspective. *Pak. Vet. J.* **32**(2): 1–9.

Adone R. and Pasquali P. (2013): Epidemio surveillance of brucellosis. *Rev. sci. tech. Off. int. Epiz.*,**32** (1): 199-205.

Afify M., Al-Zahrani S.H., and El-Koumi M.A. (2013): Brucellosis-Induced Pancytopenia in Children: *A Prospective Study. Life Sci. J.***10**:1.

African Uion-Interafrican Bureau for Animal resources, 2 September (2013): Brucellosis (*Brucella abortus*). Available at *http://www.au-ibar.org.* (Accessed on December 10, 2021).

Akhtar R., Chaudhry Z.I., Shakoori A.R., Ahmad M., and Aslam A. (2010): Comparative efficacy of conventional diagnostic methods and evaluation of polymerase chain reaction for the diagnosis of Bovine Brucellosis. *Vet. World* **3**(2): 53–56.

Aliskan, H. (2008): The value of culture and serological methods in the diagnosis of human brucellosis. *Microbiol. Bul.*, **42**:185-195.

Almuneef M. and Memish Z.A. (2003): Prevalence of Brucella antibodies after acute brucellosis. *J. Chemother.*; **15**:148-151.

Anonymous (2007): Animal Health Disease Cards. Bovine Brucellosis. Available at *http://www.fao.org/ag/againfo/subjects/en/health/diseases-cards/brucellosi-bo.html* (Accessed on *December* 6, 2021).

Araj G.F. (1999): Human brucellosis: a classical infectious disease with persistent diagnostic challenges. Clin. Lab. Sci. **12**: 207-212.

Australian Veterinary Emergency Plan (AUSVETPLAN), (2005): Bovine Brucellosis Prevalence in and around Australia. *3 rd. ed J. Applied Microbiol.*, **11**: 8-9

Baldwin C.L. and Goenka R. (2006): Host immune responses to the intracellular bacterium *Brucella*: does the bacterium instruct the host to facilitate chronic infection? *Crit. Rev.*

Barroso G.P., Rodriguez-Contreras P.R., Gil E.B., Maldonado M.A., Guijarro H.G., and Martin, S.A. (2002): Study of 1,595 brucellosis cases in the Almeria province based on epidemiological data from disease reporting. Rev. Clin. Esp., **202**:577-582.

Beker F. and Kedir U. (2008): Serology. EPHTI; Pp. 7-11.

Brinley M.J., Mackinnon D.J., Lawson J.R., and Cullen G.A. (1996): The Rose Bengal plate agglutination test in the diagnosis of brucellosis. Vet. Rec., **85**: 636-641.

Buchanan T.M. and Faber L.C. (1980): 2-Mercaptoethanol Brucella agglutination test: usefulness for predicting recovery from brucellosis. *J. Clin. Microbiol.*;**11**: 691-693.

Butler J., Seawright G., McGivern P., and Gilsdorf M. (1986): Preliminary evidence for a diagnostic Immunoglobulin G1 antibody response among culture- positive cows vaccinated with Brucella *abortus* strain 19 and challenge exposed with strain 2308. *Am. J. Vet. Res.*; **47**:1258-1264.

Campos P.C., Gomes M.T.R., Guimaraes G., Costa Franco M.M., Marim F.M., and Oliveira S.C. (2014): Brucella *abortus* DNA is a major agonist to activate the host innate immune system. Micro. Infect. **16**: 979-984.

Carrasco E.A., Uzal F.A., and Nielsen K. (1995): Comparison of four ELISA techniques in the evaluation of the serological response of heifers vaccinated with Brucella *abortus* strain 19. Arch. Med. Vet. 27 (Special Issue SI): 51-57.

Carvalho N., Mol J., Xavier M., Paixao T., Lage A., and Santos A. (2010): 'Pathogenesis of Bovine Brucellosis', *vet. j.*, **184**(2): 146-155

Chimana H.M., Muma J.B., Samui K.L., Hangombe B.M., Munyeme M., Matope G., Phiri A.M., Skjerve E., and Tryland M. (2010): A comparative study of the seroprevalence of brucellosis in commercial and small–scale mixed dairy beef cattle enterprises of Lusaka province and Chibombo district, Zambia. Trop. Anim. Health Prod. **42**(7): 1541–1545.

Cho D., Nam H., Kim J., Heo E., Cho Y., Hwang I., Kim J., Kim J., and Jung S. (2010): Quantative Rose Bengal Test for diagnosis of Bovine Brucellosis. *J. Immunoassay Immunochem.*;**31** (2): 120-130.

Christopher S., Umapathy B.L., and Ravikumar K. L. (2010): Brucellosis: review on the recent trends in pathogenicity and laboratory diagnosis. *J. Lab. Phys.* **2**(2):55–60.

Clavijo E., Díaz R., Anguita Á., García A. Pinedo A. and Smits H.L. (2003): Comparison of a Dipstick Assay for Detection of Brucella-Specific Immunoglobulin M Antibodies with Other Tests for Serodiagnosis of Human Brucellosis. Clin Diagn Lab Immunol, **10**:612-615.

Corbel M.J. and MacMillan A. (2000): Bovine Brucellosis. In "Manual of standards for diagnostic tests and vaccines". Office International des Epizooties. Paris.

Corbel M.J., Garin-Bastuji B., Díaz R., Young E. (2006): Brucellosis in humans and animals. WHO Press, Pp. 12. ISBN: 9241547138.

Crowther J.R. (2010): The ELISA guidebook. 2nd (ed.), Method in Molecular Biology. Humana press Totowa, New Jersey, USA.

Di Febo T., Luciani M., Portanti O., Bonfini B., Lelli R., and Tittarelli M. (2012): Development and evaluation of diagnostic tests for the serological diagnosis of brucellosis in swine. *Veterinaria Italiana*, v. 48, n. 2, Pp. 145-156.

Díaz R., Casanova A., Ariza J., and Moriyón I. (2011): The Rose Bengal Test in human brucellosis: a neglected test for the diagnosis of a neglected disease. *PLoS. Negl. Trop. Dis.***5**: 950.Available at*http://www.ncbi.nlm.nih.gov/pubmed/17792012*

Dranoff G. (2004): Cytokines in cancer pathogenesis and cancer therapy. Nat. Rev. Cancer, **4**(1):11-22

Enoe C., Georgiadis M., and Johnson W. (2000): 'Estimation of sensitivity and specificity of diagnostic tests and disease prevalence when the true disease state is unkown'. *Prev. Med.,***45**(1-2): 61-81.

Ertek M., Yazgi H., Ozkurt Z., Ayyildiz A., and Parlak M. (2006): Comparison of the diagnostic value of the standard Tube Agglutination Test and the ELISA IgG and IgM in patients with Brucellosis. *Turk J. Med Sci.* **36**(3):159-163.

Esmaeilzadeh A. (2004): ELISA vs. routine tests in the diagnosis of patients with brucellosis. 14th European Congress of Clinical Microbiology and Infectious Disease. Prague/Czech Republic, Abstract number: 903_r2158, May 1–4.

European Commission (2009): Working document on eradication of bovine, sheep and goats brucellosis in the European Union accepted by the "bovine" and "sheep and goats" brucellosis subgroups of the Task Force on monitoring animal disease eradication. Pp. 6-7

FAO (2003): Guidelines for coordinated human and animal brucellosis surveillance. FAO Animal Production and Health Paper Pp.; 156.

FAO (2005): Bovine Brucellosis. retired 24 *December* 2021 from http://www.fao.org/ag/againfo/subjects/en/health/diseases-cards/brucellosi-bo.html

Fernando P.P., Klaus N., Luis E., S. and Wei L. Y. (2010): Diagnosis of Brucellosis. *The Open Vet. Sci. J.* **4**: 46-60.

Foster J.T., Okinaka R.T., Svensson R., Shaw K., De B.K., Robison R.A., Probert W.S., Kenefic L.J., Brown W.D., and Keim P. (2008): Real-time PCR assays of single-nucleotide polymorphisms defining the major Brucella clades. *J. Clin. Microbiol.*,**46**: 296–301.

Galinska E.M. and Zagorski J. (2013): Brucellosis in humans, etiology, diagnostics, clinical forms. *Ann. Agric. Environ. Med.* **20**(2):233.245

Giambartolomei G., Zwerdling A., Cassataro J., Bruno L., Fossati C., and Philipp M. (2004): Lipoproteins, not lipopolysaccharide, are the key mediators of the pro-inflammatoryresponse elicited by heat-killed *Brucella abortus*. *J.Immunol.* **173**(7):4635-4642.

Godfroid J. (2002): Brucellosis in wildlife. Rev Sci Tech.; **21**:277–286.

Goenka R., Guirnalda P.D., Black S.J., and Baldwin C.L. (2012): B lymphocytes provide an infection niche for intracellular bacterium *Brucella abortus*. *J. Infect Dis.*,**206**(1):9

Greiner M. and Gardner I. (2000): 'Epidemiological issues in the validation of veterinary diagnostic tests', prev. med., **45**(1-2): 3-22.

Greiner M., Verloo D., and de Massis F. (2009): Meta-analytical equivalence studies on diagnostic tests for Bovine Brucellosis allowing assessment of a test against a group of comparative tests. Prev. Vet. Med.; **92**:373-381

Gupte S. and Kaur T. (2015): Diagnosis of Human Brucellosis. *J. Trop. Dis.*, **4**:1

Hatami H., Soori A., Janbakhsh R., and Mansouri F. (2010): Epidemiological, clinical, and laboratory features of brucellar meningitis. Arch. Iran Med., **13**: 486-491.

He Y. (2012): "Analyses of Brucella Pathogenesis, Host Immunity, and Vaccine Targets Using Systems Biology and Bioinformatics," Frontiers in Cellular and Infection Microbiology,Vol. 2, Pp. 2. *Immunol.*,**26**: 407-442.

Janeway.charles.travers(2001):Immunobiology(5th ed), newyork:garland science, ISBNO-8153-3642-X retired 24 *December* 2021.

Jarvis B.W., Harris T.H., Qureshi N., and Splitter G.A. (2002): Rough lipopolysaccharide from Brucella *abortus* and Escherichia coli differentially activates the same mitogen-activated protein kinase signaling pathways for tumor necrosis factor alpha in RAW 264.7 macrophage-like cells. Infect. Immun. **70**: 7165-7168

Joint FAO/WHO Expert Committee on Brucellosis (1986): Sixth Report of a joint FAO/WHO expert committee on brucellosis, Technical ReportSeries 740, WHO, Geneva, Switzerland.

Kaufmann S.H. (1999): Cell-mediated immunity: dealing a direct blow to pathogens. Curr Biol. 9:97-99.

Kolar J., (1984): Diagnosis and Control of Brucellosis in Small Ruminants. Prev. Vet. Med. 2:215-225.

Konstantinidis A., Minas A., Pournaras S., Kansouzidou A., Papastergiu P., Maniatis A., Stathatis N., and Hadjichristodoulou C. (2007): Evaluation and comparison of fluorescence polarization assay with three of the currently used serological tests in diagnosis of human brucellosis. J. Clin. Microbiol. Inect. Dis., 26: 715-721.

Kostoula A., Bobogianni H., Virioni G., and Tabatabai L.B. (2001): Detection of Brucella IgG, IgM and IgA antibodies with ELISA method in patients with Brucellosis. Clin. Microbiol. Infect. 7(1):108-1058.

Lucero N. E., Ayala S.M., Escobar G.I., and Jacob N.R. (2007): The value of serologic tests for diagnosis and follow up of patients having brucellosis. Am. J. Infect. Dis., 3: 27–35.

Mantur B.G., Birada M.S., Bidri R.C., Mulimani M.S., and Kariholu P. (2006): Protean clinical manifestations and diagnostic challenges of human brucellosis in adults: 16 years' experience in an endemic area. J. Med. Microbiol.;55:897-903.

Martirosyan A. and Gorvel J.P. (2013): Brucella evasion of adaptive immunity. Future Microbiol. 8: 147-154.

McGiven J. A., Tucker J. D., Perrett L. L., Stack J. A., Brew S.D., and MacMillan A.P. (2003): "Validation of FPA and cELISA for the Detection of Antibodies to Brucella abortus in Cattle Sera and Comparison to SAT, CFT, and iELISA," J. Immunol. Methods, Vol. 278, No. 1-2, Pp. 171-178.

Mcnaught D.J., Chappel R.J., Allan G.S., Bourke J.A., and Rogerson B.A. (1977): The effects of IgG2 and of antigen concentration on prozoning in the complement fixation test for Bovine Brucellosis. Res. Vet. Sci. (in the Press).

Miguel J.D., Marín C.M., Mun P.M., Dieste O.L., Grillo´M.J., and Blasco J.M. (2011): Development of a Selective Culture Medium for Primary Isolation of the Main Brucella Species. J. clin. Microbial. Pp.;1458-1463.

Montagnaro S., Longo M., Mallardo K., and *Lovane G.* (2008): Evaluation of fluorescence polarization assay for the detection of serum antibodies to *Brucella abortus* in water buffalo (*Bubalus bubalis*). Vet.Immunol. Immunopathol.;**125**: 135-142.

Montagnaro S., Pagnini U., Diana T., Bruno L., Baldi L., and Iovane G. (2007): Comparison of fluorescence polarization assay with Rose Bengal test and complement fixation tests for the diagnosis of buffalo (Bubalus bubalis) brucellosis in a high-prevalence area. *It. J. An. Sci.*, 6:sup2, 858-861, DOI: 10.4081/ijas. 2007.s2.858.

Morgan WJ, MacKinnon DJ, Lawson JR, Cullen GA. (1969): Rose Bengal plate agglutination test in the diagnosis of brucellosis. **85**:636-641.

Munoz P., Marin C., Monreal D., Gonzales D., Garin-Bastuji B., Diaz R., Mainar-Jaime R., Moriyon I., and Blasco J. (2005): Efficacy of several serological tests and antigens for the diagnosis of Bovine Brucellosis in the presence of false positive serological results due to *Yersinia enterocolitica* O:9. *Clin. Diagn. Lab. Immunol.*, **12**: 141-151.

Muriuki S.M., McDermott J.J., Arimi S.M., Mugambi J.T., and Wamola I.A. (1997): Criteria for better detection of brucellosis in the Narok District of Kenya. *East Afr. Med. J.* **74**: 317–320.

Nauseef W.M. (2007): How human neutrophils kill and degrade microbes: an integrated view. *Immunol. Rev.*, **219**: 88-102.

Nicoletti P. and Fincher M.G. (1966): The recovery of Brucella *abortus* strain 19-like organism. Cornell Vet, **56**:167-171.

Nicoletti P.L. (1990): Vaccination. In: Nielsen KH and Duncan JR (eds). Animal Brucellosis. CRC Press, Boca Raton, Pp, 283-299

Nielsen K., Gall D., Jolley M., Leishman G., Balsevicus S., Smith P., Nicoletti P., and Thomas F. (1996): A homogeneous fluorescence polarization antibody assay for detection of antibody to Brucella *abortus*. *J. Immunol. Methods*.**195**: 161-168

Nielsen K. (2002): Diagnosis of brucellosis by serology. Vet. Microbiol.,**90**: 447-459.

Noriello S. (2004): Laboratory-acquired brucellosis-Detection of *Brucella abortus* in Bovine Milk by Polymerase Chain Reaction. Emerg. Infect. Dis., **10**:1848-1850.

OIE (2000): Ovine Epididimytis (B. *Ovis*). Manual of standard for Diagnostic Test and Vaccines. 3rd ed. OIE, Paris, France, 467-474.

OIE (2004): Bovine Brucellosis. Section 2.3 in OIE manual of Standards for diagnostic tests and vaccines. 5th ed. OIE Paris.

OIE (2008): Bovine Brucellosis. In: Manual of Diagnostic Tests and Vaccines for Terrestrial Animals, CHAPTER 2.4.3. [Online] http://www.oie.int/fr/normes/mmanual/2008/pdf/2.04.03. Bovine Brucell.pdf [consulted 8 *December* 2021a].

OIE (2009): Chapter 2.4.3. Bovine Brucellosis OIE Terrestrial Manual.chapter,05/222012. http://www.oie. Int/international-standard-seeting/Terrestrial Manual/access online/accessed on 8 *December* 2021.

OIE (2013): principles and methods of validation of diagnostic assays for infectious disease, 03/052015

Oliveira S.C., Soeurt N., and Splitter G.A., (2002): Molecular and cellular interactions between Brucella *abortus* antigens and host immune responses. Vet. Microbiol. **90**: 417-424.

Orduna A., Almaraz A., Prado A., Gutierrez M.P., García-Pascual A., Dueñas A., Cuervo M., Abad R., Hernández B., Lorenzo B., Bratos M.A., and Rodrígueztorres A. (2000): Evaluation of an immunocapture-agglutination test 84 (Brucellacapt) for the seodiagnosis of human brucellosis. *J. Clin. Microbiol.* **38**:4000-4005.

Parent M.A., Goenka R., Murphy E., Levier K., Carreiro N., Golding B., Ferguson G., Roop R.M., Walker G.C., and Baldwin C.L. (2007): *Brucella abortus* bac A mutant induces greater pro-inflammatory cytokines than the wild-type parents train. *Micro. Infect.* **9**: 55–62.

Parkin J. and Cohen B. (2001): An overview of the immune system. Lancet, **357**(9270):1777-1789.

Pasquevich K., García Samartino C., Coria L., Estein S., Zwerdling A., Ibañez A., Barrionuevo P., Oliveira F., Carvalho N., Borkowski J., Oliveira S., Warzecha H., Giambartolomei G., and Cassataro J. (2010): The protein moiety of Brucella *abortus* outer membrane protein 16 is a new bacterial pathogen-associated molecular pattern that activates dendritic cells in vivo, induces a Th1 immune response, and is a promising self-adjuvating vaccine against systemic and oral acquired brucellosis. *J. Immunol.*, 184(9):5200-5212.

Paulo P., Vigliocco A., Ramondino R., Marticorena D., Bissi E., Briones G., Gorchs C., Gall D., and Nielsen K. (2000): Evaluation of primary binding assays for the presumptive serodiagnosis of swine brucellosis in Argentina. Clin. Diagn. Lab. Immunol.; **7**: 828-831.

Perrett L.L., McGiven J.A., Brew S.D., and Stack J.A. (2010): Evaluation of competitive ELISA for detection of antibodies to Brucella infection in domestic animals. *Croatian Medical J.*, v.51, n. 4, Pp. 314-319.

Plackett P. and Alton, G.G. (1975): A mechanism for prozone formation in the complement fixation test for Bovine Brucellosis. *Aust. Vet. J.* **51**:374.

Pouillot R., Garin-Bastuji B., Gerbier G., Coche Y., Cau C., Dufour B., and Moutou F. (1997): The brucellin skin test as a tool to differentiate false positive serological reactions in bovine brucellosis. Vet.Res.,**28**:365-374.

Radostits E. D., Gay C. C., and Inchcliff W. K. (2000): Veterinary Medicine, Textbook of the Diseases of Cattle, Sheep, Pigs, Goats and Horses. 9th ed., New York, W.B. Saunders Company Ltd, Pp: 867-882.

Roushan M.R., Amin M.J., Abdoel T.H., and Smits H.L. (2005): Application of a user-friendly Brucella-specific IgM and IgG antibody assay for the rapid confirmation of Rose Bengal positive patients in a hospital in Iran. *Trans. R. Soc. rop. Med. Hyg.* **99**(10):744-750.

Ryan K.J., Ray C.G., eds. (2004): Sherris Medical Microbiology (4[th]ed.). McGraw Hill. Pp. 247–249. ISBN 0-8385-8529-9.

Saegerman C., Vo T., De Waele L., Gilson D., Bastin A., D*ubray G.,* Flanagan P., Limet J.,Letesson J., and Godfroid J. (1999): Diagnosis of Bovine Brucellosis by skin test: conditions for the test and evaluation of its performance. Vet. Rec. **145**: 214-218.

Salama Abdel Hafez M.A., Khaled A. A. Hany M. H., and Ibrahim G. (2011): Comparative diagnosis of ovine brucellosis using single step blood-PCR with old and new serological tools. *African J.Microbiol.Res.*;**5**(23):3976-3980.

Samartino L., Gall D., Gregoret R., Nielsen K. (1999): Validation of enzyme-linked immunosorbent assays for the diagnosis of Bovine Brucellosis. Vet. Microbiol.;**70**: 193-200.

Schelling E., Diguimbaye C., Daoud S., Nicolet J., Boerlin P., TannerM., and Zinsstag J. (2003): Brucellosis and Q-fever sero-prevalence of nomadic pastoralists and their livestock in Chad. Prev. Vet. Med.; **61**: 279-293.

Serra J. and Vinas M. (2004): Laboratory diagnosis of brucellosis in a rural endemic area in northeastern Spain. *Int. Microbiol.,* 7(1):53–58.

Skendros P,Boura p.(2013): Immunity to brucellosis.Rev Sci Tech. 32(1):137-147

Steingart K.R., Ramsay A., Dowdy D.W., and Pai M. (2012): Serological tests for the diagnosis of active tuberculosis: relevance for India. *Indian J. Med. Res.*135, Pp 695-702.

Supriya C., Umapathy B.L., and Ravikumar K.L. (2010): Brucellosis: review on the recent trends in pathogenicity and laboratory diagnosis. *J. Lab. Physicians*2: 55-60.

Thompson I., McGiven J., Sawyer J., Thirlwall R., Commander N., and Stack J. (2009): Competitive electrochemiluminescence wash and no-wash immunoassays for detection of serum antibodies to smooth Brucella strains. Clin. Vaccine Immunol.; **16**: 765-771.1999; **6**: 269-272.

Tigard I.R. (2012): Veterinary Immunology an Introduction. 9th ed. Sounders, Philadelphia, Pp. 61-74.

Tigard I.R. (2013): Veterinary Immunology, 9th ed. Pp. 3-5.

World Health Organization (1971): Joint FAO/WHO Expert Committee on Brucellosis, 5th report. WHO Technical Report Series No. 464.

Wright P.F., Tounkar A.K., Lelent A.M., and Jeggo M.H. (1997): International reference Standards: antibody standards for the indirect enzyme-linked immunosorbent assay. Rev. Sci. Tech., **3**:824-832.

Xavler M.N., T.A. Palxao, E.P. Poester, A.P. Lage and Santos R.L. (2009): Pathology, immunohistochemistry and bacteriology of tissues and milk of cows and fetuses experimentally infected with Brucella *abortus. J. Comp. Pathol.*, **140**: 147-157.

Young EJ. (2005): Brucella species. In: Mandell G.L., Douglas R.G., Bennett J.E., and Dolin R., editors. Mandell, Douglas and Bennett's. principles and practice of infectious diseases. New York: Churchill Livingstone; Pp. 2669-2674.

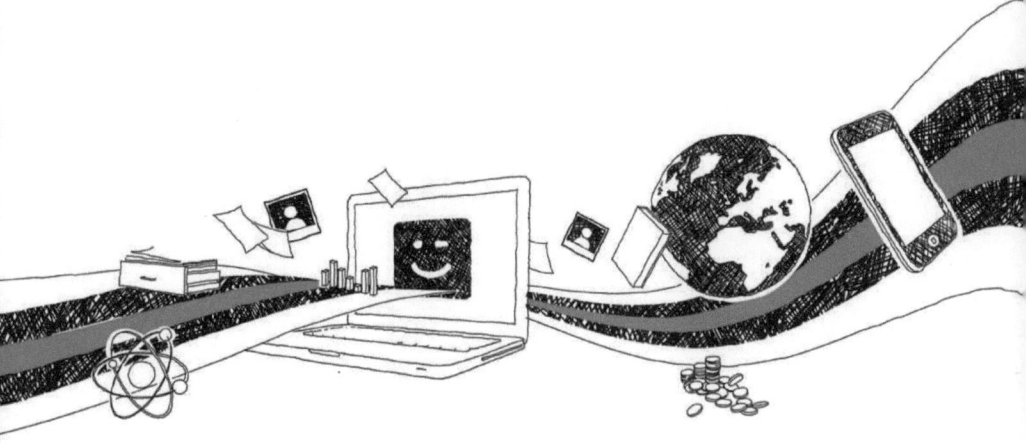
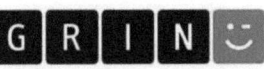